Individual Service Funds

a guide to making Self-Directed Support work for everyone

by **Sam Smith and Frances Brown on behalf of In Control Scotland**

Published by the Centre for Welfare Reform
in association with Citizen Network

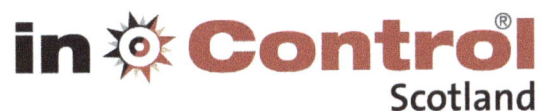

in ☀ Control® Scotland

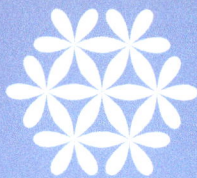

Publishing information

Individual Service Funds © Sam Smith and Frances Brown 2018
Figures 1, 2, and 3 © Simon Duffy 2018

Designed by Henry Iles
First published February 2018
ISBN print: 978–1–907790–95–9
36 pp.

Individual Service Funds is published by the Centre for Welfare Reform.

The publication is free to download from:
www.centreforwelfarereform.org

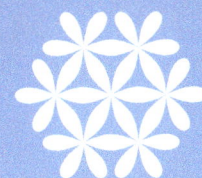

Contents

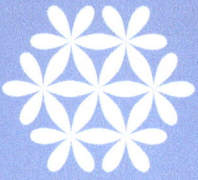

Foreword

The use of an Individual Service Fund as a way that people can have more control, choice and flexibility in their support is not a new idea. In Scotland, Individual Service Funds have been used by a small number of organisations for more than 20 years as a way to enable people to take more control over their life and their support, even if they were not deemed to have the capacity to take a Direct Payment. The authors of this paper have a long standing commitment to this approach and can describe clearly how an Individual Service Fund works and why it makes Self-Directed Support available for everyone.

This paper was commissioned by In Control Scotland with the aim of promoting inclusion and social justice through greater understanding of the benefits of the creative use of Individual Service Funds. It is intended to be an enabling document which will be of value to individuals, families, care providers and funders. It is intended to inspire greater consideration of the untapped transformational potential of Individual Service Funds by providing lived examples. It also takes the form of a provocation, intended to stimulate questions and conversations about where power, choice and control lie in any situation involving an individual budget.

Individual Service Funds, as described in this paper, are rooted in a human rights based approach, drawing on the aspirations articulated in the *UN Convention on the Rights of Persons with Disabilities* (UNCRPD), the legal framework of the *European Convention on Human Rights* (ECHR) and making a practical reality of the Scottish Government *PANEL* principles.[1,2,3] This paper should also be read alongside the *Fair Work Convention* with it's stated commitment to fair work practices as a means to drive success, wellbeing and prosperity for individuals, businesses, organisations and society.[4]

We believe that there is still a lot more that can be done to make Self-Directed Support work for everyone and that greater use of Individual Service Funds as described in this paper is one way to unlocking its potential. We hope that you enjoy reading, thinking about and discussing this document and the ideas and experiences contained in it.

Keith Etherington
In Control Scotland

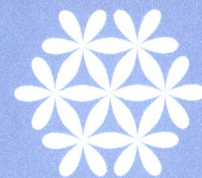

Introduction

An Individual Service Fund (ISF) is one way of managing an individual budget available under Option 2 of the Social Care (Self-Directed Support) (Scotland) Act 2013.[5] The ideas and values underpinning Self-Directed Support draw deeply on disabled people's activism. Particularly the hard-fought struggle to develop Direct Payments as a mechanism to gain greater choice and control over their support arrangement and the way it is organised.[6]

These ideas are not only relevant to Scotland. Similar approaches are found in England and in other countries using Self-Directed Support around the world. They are similar to what is known as *Shared Management* in Australia.

This paper outlines the core components of an ISF. It details what needs to be in place for an ISF to work for all the partners involved.

It also provides a framework by which to measure whether an ISF arrangement is creative and flexible enough to assist a person to achieve their outcomes for a good life and not just a service.

Lived examples of the creative uses of individual budgets help to illustrate how ISFs can provide the choice and control of a Direct Payment, without the need to take on the full responsibility of becoming an employer.

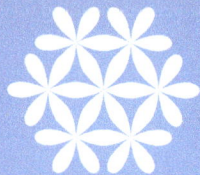

Background

ISFs were first used in Scotland by Inclusion Glasgow in 1996 in order to offer people the choice and control associated with a Direct Payment without the workload associated with becoming an employer.[7] Subsequently this approach was adopted by other organisations and with the introduction of the Social Care (Self-Directed Support) (Scotland) Act 2013, has become a formally validated mechanism for managing an individual budget.[8]

There are a range of options available under the Act, to ensure everyone can exercise choice and control over their support arrangement:

- Option 1: A Direct Payment (a cash payment)
- Option 2: Funding allocated to a provider of choice or other third party
- Option 3: The council can arrange a service
- Option 4: A mix of these options for different types of support

An ISF is the practical mechanism that enables you to select Option 2. With Option 2 you not only get to choose who provides you with support, but also you get to work with your chosen support provider to make flexible and creative use of your individual budget.

Independent Living

The purpose of Option 2 is to enable you to enjoy your human right to independent living. For as the statutory guidance to accompany the Social Care (Self-Directed Support) (Scotland) Act 2013 states:

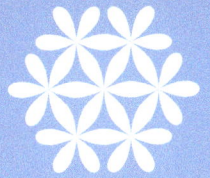

Independent living means all disabled people having the same freedom, choice, dignity and control as other citizens at home, work and in the community. It does not necessarily mean living by yourself or fending for yourself. It means rights to practical assistance and support to participate in society and live an ordinary life.[9]

Figure 1 illustrates that, whatever option an individual adopts to direct their support arrangement, the orientation should be towards the 'North Star' of independent living. Choosing to take a Direct Payment gives an individual the ultimate choice and control over how they organise and receive support. Choosing Option 2, and using an ISF as illustrated in this paper, should offer the same choice and control, but without the need to take full responsibility for managing the money or becoming an employer.

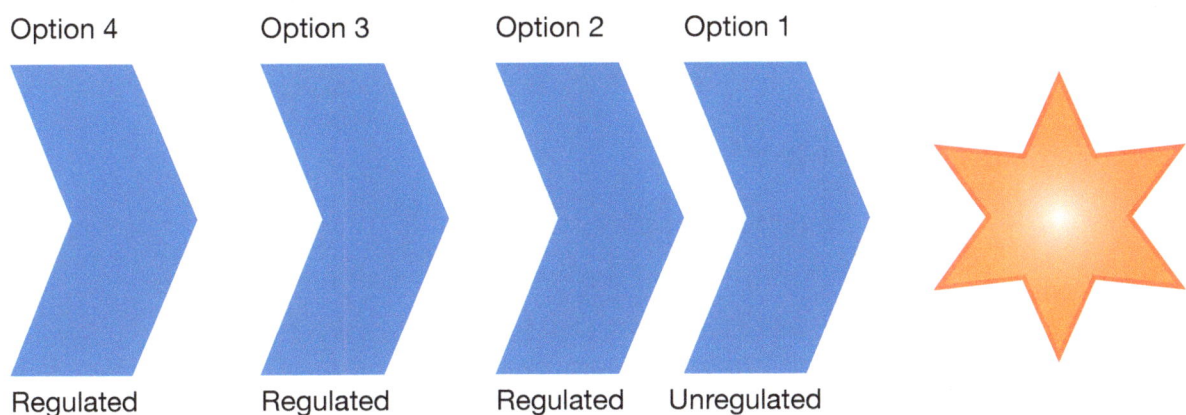

Option 4	Option 3	Option 2	Option 1	
Regulated	Regulated	Regulated	Unregulated	

FIGURE 1. THE GOAL OF THE SELF DIRECTED SUPPORT OPTIONS

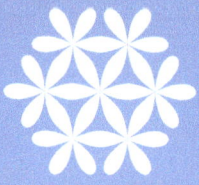

ISFs work for anyone regardless of age, support needs, diagnoses, mental capacity or legal status. ISFs provide the capacity for support to flex and change as required; this can be particularly beneficial for individuals experiencing fluctuating health conditions. ISFs also ensure that appropriate checks and balances are in place to support choice and control for individuals who may struggle to make decisions or have difficulty managing risk. ISFs provide a safe and supportive mechanism to ensure that more people can benefit from Self-Directed Support. Importantly an ISF is a mechanism for managing an individual budget to live a good life not just to receive a service.

What is an Individual Service Fund?

An ISF is a way of managing an individual budget so as to support a person to achieve their identified outcomes, ensuring they can live the life they aspire to. The language of Self-Directed Support can be confusing and sometimes it can appear that new words are being used to describe familiar practices. We have identified four distinct components of an ISF which should help clarify what makes them important:

To qualify as an ISF there needs to be:

1. An **upfront individual budget** allocation
2. A **flexible support** arrangement designed around the person
3. A budget that is used to **focus on a good life** not just a service
4. **Maximum control** for the person over decision making

These four elements mirror the choice and control that is available to an individual who has opted to select a Direct Payment. In the next section of this paper we describe the general principles underlying each of these four components. This will be followed by some questions you may ask if you are unsure whether you are working with an ISF.

Upfront individual budget

Flexible support

Focus on a good life

Maximum control

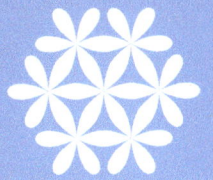

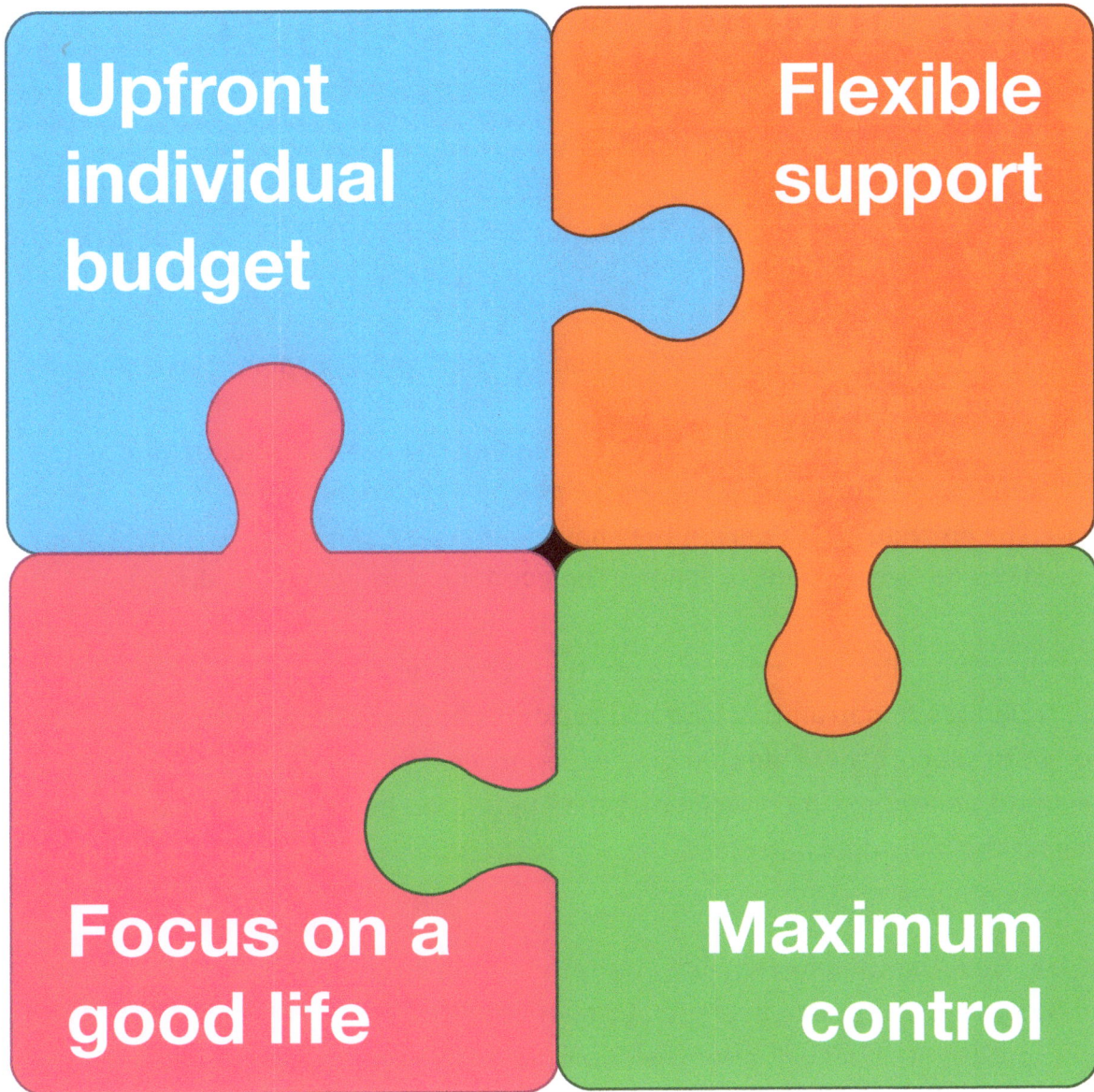

FIGURE 2. KEY COMPONENTS OF AN ISF

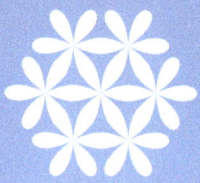

1. Upfront individual budget

For an individual budget to be managed using an ISF there needs to be an explicit allocation of funding ring fenced for the person. This may take the form of an annual budget or a fixed allocation for a shorter-term need.

- **The amount of money must be clear, up front and transparent so that it can inform the planning process.**
- **It does not matter how the level of funding has been agreed, so long as the amount is sufficient to achieve the person's stated outcomes.**
- **The individual, or a person they have nominated, should be in control of how their budget is spent to achieve the good life they wish to lead.**

Lives are not predictable, events happen that we cannot foresee, health improves or deteriorates, opportunities arise and accidents happen. An ISF should be flexible enough to support these life changing experiences, enabling increases and decreases in support as required. It is crucial that the budget can be used in whatever way best achieves the individual outcomes; the only restriction should be that the activity or purchase is legal.

The ISF should be used to enhance, strengthen and support existing relationships and connections not place bureaucratic restrictions in the way of a good life. It is also important that the individual, or their nominated person, receives regular routine financial feedback on the way their budget is being spent. This should be in an accessible form that enables the individual to know, understand and make informed decisions about their budget and any changes they may like to make.

General Principles:

- There is an explicit upfront allocation of funding ring fenced for the person.
- The budget informs the planning process.
- The person (or nominated other i.e. family member) is in control of how the budget is used to achieve their desired outcomes.

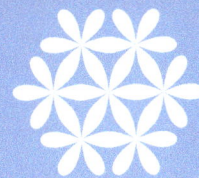

- The support arrangement is flexible and changes as the individuals' life changes.
- There are no restrictions on how the budget is used as long as it helps to achieve the person's outcomes and any necessary action is legal.
- Regular updates are available on how the budget is being used and what has been achieved with it.

Maureen, David and Freddie

Freddie was a 9 year old boy who lived at home with his parents Maureen and David, who both worked full time. Freddie had a wide range of complex health conditions and his mum and dad looked after him full time outwith school hours. Traditional respite services had not worked well and had resulted in Freddie being hospitalised. Maureen and David felt unable to take on the additional responsibility of a Direct Payment. The local authority identified a small individual budget (less than £10,000) and, with the assistance of a support provider, they came up with a plan detailing what would make the most difference to them as a family.

1. Freddie was doubly incontinent, this meant the washing machine was on constantly and the house was always noisy. They opted to pay for a weekly laundry uplift service. This relieved them of some of the repetitive heavy chores, the house was calmer and quieter and Freddie was more content.

2. They paid for the airfare and accommodation for a family member to support them on a short family break to Disneyland Paris.

3. Two Personal Assistants (PAs), who lived locally, were recruited and then trained by David, Maureen and health professionals in how to support Freddie. Twice a week the PAs would be at home waiting for Freddie to arrive on the school bus. This allowed David and Maureen to go shopping after work, go to routine appointments and take part in other activities.

A relatively small budget, used flexibly, transformed day to day life for Freddie and his parents.

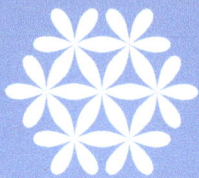

What to expect if you have chosen Option 2 and are using an ISF:

- You know the individual budget allocation upfront before you start planning.
- You are involved in planning how to spend your budget.
- You get regular updates on how your budget is being spent.
- You choose how things are organised and how this affects your budget.

What an organisation must have in place if they are offering ISFs:

- Facility to manage the person's individual budget.
- Capacity to support people to plan creatively using their individual budgets.
- Ability to routinely report to the person on how their budget has been spent and what it has achieved.
- Flexibility to change the support arrangement as the person's life changes.

What commissioners must have in place if they are funding an ISF:

- A transparent system for the allocation of the annual individual budget.
- The ability to let people know their budget allocation upfront.
- A clear and simple process for agreeing a plan for a good life incorporating agreed outcomes and a budget.
- Transparent, least restrictive, rules about how a budget can be spent.
- Systems and contracts that allow plans to change quickly and give people the flexibility to respond to life as it changes.

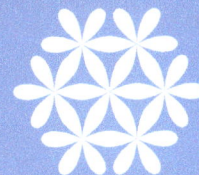

Helen and Dan

Helen was advised of her son Dan's individual budget allocation. Initially Helen did not believe the allocation was enough to meet her son's needs as Dan needed some support to be provided by two staff. Helen asked the social worker to challenge the allocation, the local authority restated that the allocation was fair.

Helen embraced the planning process and, with the help of an independent facilitator, considered how the money could be used to achieve her son's desired outcomes and achieve a better life. Together they reshaped Dan's support so that made more sense for Dan and Helen. The allocated budget provided for the direct support required plus it also enabled the purchase of a bespoke bed which also made life easier and safer for Dan and Helen.

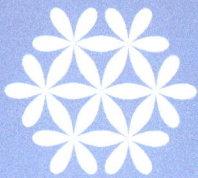

2. Flexible support

The purpose of an ISF is to enable a person to actively participate in the creation of a support arrangement that suits their individual needs and lifestyle.

- The design of a support arrangement should consider a person's skills, gifts and aspirations as well as the areas of their life where they may need additional support.
- It should also take into account the wide range of assets and resources available within existing relationships and within the wider community.
- Crucially the person should be at the heart of the discussion, the planning and the design. A plan can only make sense as a way forward if it makes sense to the person.

The flexibility of an ISF should allow people to try things out, make mistakes, change their mind and learn from each of these opportunities. An ISF must enable the support arrangement to change as the person's life changes.

The rules around the use of an ISF need to be transparent and simple enough so that everyone understands and knows where they stand. The person must be given the freedom and flexibility to apply creative solutions to sometimes complex, emotional and intimate situations. We advocate a very simple rule of thumb, if it meets an agreed outcome, doesn't harm anyone or place a person at unreasonable risk and it's legal it should happen.

If a person chooses to work with a service provider, they should able to tailor the support they receive in a way that makes sense for them. The cost of any service provided should be clear and transparent; this does not mean it needs to be broken down into an hourly rate. Many of the services we value are not broken down into hours, nor do they use hourly rates. A visit to the hairdresser, a meal in a restaurant, a

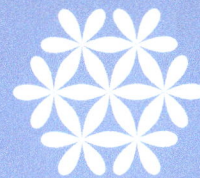

visit to the dentist, surgical procedures are all assessed on the outcome they achieve, not on how long it took and what it cost by the hour. It is important for a person to know what outcome they want to achieve and what this may cost.

Support arrangements designed using an ISF should focus on every day, community-based and mainstream options, in addition to specialist services. The purpose of an ISF is to ensure that the person at the heart of the plan has choice and control over the support arrangement, the purpose of which is for them to remain healthy and well and live a good life.

General Principles:

- Having an ISF means that people don't fit into services, they have the kind of support that suits them, when they want it.
- The starting point for service design should be consideration of the individual's skills, gifts and aspirations, their assets and the resources available to them in their existing relationships and community.
- The person must always be at the heart of the thinking, planning and doing.
- Support must change as the person's life changes.
- The person can use their individual budget to access a range of additional resources.
- If the person uses the money to purchase the services of a provider organisation they should have the opportunity to tailor how they get their support, in a way that makes sense to them.
- Costs for services must be clear and transparent.
- The service designed for each person should be tailored to them, be creative and offer the chance to use ordinary, everyday solutions as well as specialist supports.
- Every service design and plan must support the person to remain healthy, safe and well.

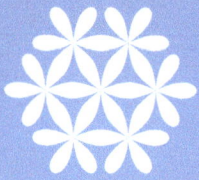

Kenny

Kenny was a young man with mental health and addiction issues that has resulted in him spending long periods of time in inpatient units. Kenny, and those who knew and cared about him, had lost sight of what his good life might look like. All the focus was on the problems and difficulties he experienced. Kenny was allocated an individual budget and this was used to plan with Kenny, his family and multi-agency colleagues with a focus on what a good life might look like. Having identified this, realising it became the goal that everyone worked towards.

Kenny moved out of hospital and into the first home of his own. With only one setback, when he briefly returned to the unit, Kenny's life has transformed. His level of direct support has reduced as he wants time and space to enjoy the privacy of his home. His focus is now on gaining paid employment and he is using part of his individual budget to set up a micro enterprise. Kenny's use of his ISF has changed as his life has developed.

What to expect if you have chosen Option 2 and are using an ISF:

- You can negotiate with the organisation to tailor the support that is right for you.
- You know the cost of the supports and services on offer and these are clear and easy to understand.
- The support arrangement is planned and designed by spending time with you and people who know you and finding out what makes sense for you.
- You are as involved as much as you want to be in deciding who works for you and how things are managed.
- The organisation is flexible and responds to changes in your life and your needs, you don't need to just 'fit in'.

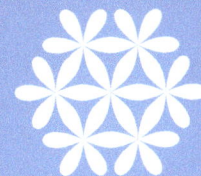

What an organisation must have in place if they are offering ISFs:

- Clarity about what they can and cannot offer.
- Transparency about all the costs attached to the services they provide.
- Capacity for personalised planning and service design.
- Recruitment and employment processes that are personalised.
- Flexibility to respond quickly and appropriately to the person's life changes.
- Creativity to work with individuals and families and about different ways of doing things.
- Facility to identify each person's ISF and systems to track how it is spent.
- Ability to routinely report to the person on how their budget has been spent and what has been achieved.
- Ability to think creatively and draw on resources outwith its own organisation.
- Resources to ensure an ongoing process for planning with people, budgeting and changing things with people as their life changes.

What commissioners must have in place if they are funding an ISF:

- An awareness of the connection between how the budget is used and the personal outcomes achieved.
- Flexibility and a reasonable measured response to changes in people's lives, their outcomes, plans and how money is spent to achieve this.
- Systems and processes that support individualised recruitment and contracts of employment.
- Providers that support people to draw up service designs that are creative and flexible, clearly detailing proposed outcomes and how these are to be met using the ISF.
- Assurance that the safety and wellbeing of the person is explicitly addressed.

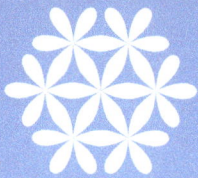

Sue and Liam

Sue and Liam are a mother and adult son who live together in their family home. Sue has a degenerative health condition and Liam has a learning disability. Sue's mother (Liam's grandmother) Patricia provided a lot of help and support to both Sue and Liam who also received support from a provider organisation.

They both had ISFs which they used to organise their own individual support arrangements. Initially Sue had very little support and Liam had a more expensive and intensive support arrangement. Over time the support arrangements changed and developed as their lives evolved.

Liam became more independent and had a reduced need for paid support whilst Sue's health deteriorated and her support changed to reflect this. Following Patricia's death, the level of informal and family support reduced significantly raising concerns about the sustainability of their support arrangement.

During a planning session Liam's skills in caring for and supporting his mother were acknowledged. This was a role he was both good at and enjoyed. The supports were reorganised to reflect this change and both Sue and Liam's ISFs were used flexibly to support this new arrangement.

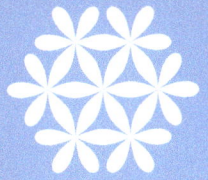

3. Focus on a good life

Many of the most important things in life cannot be bought: love, health, friendship, trust, happiness... the list goes on. That said, money, in the form of an individual budget, can make life significantly easier for people with additional support needs. It is however important to recognise that an individual budget (whether or not it's managed through an ISF) should be used for the person to achieve a good life - not just to purchase a service. It should help individuals to have higher aspirations and assist then in getting the help they need to achieve this.

The financial challenges experienced by funding authorities, taken alongside the very positive fact that people are living longer, mean that traditional approaches to service provision are neither meeting the needs of individuals, nor are they affordable in the long term. Traditional services have tended to regard those who make use of services as 'passive recipients of support' who have things done to them to meet some assessed need. ISFs provide the opportunity to co-create a support arrangement that works for each unique individual.

ISFs also harness the opportunity to draw on a far wider range of resources and opportunities that exist within the persons' own skills and gifts, within their families, neighbourhoods and communities at large. This enables creative thinking beyond what 'service land' can offer. It is important that plans for a good life draw on the widest range of resources and clearly detail how the person's individual budget will be used to achieve their desired outcomes. For the purposes of accountability, to the funding authority and for the public purse, it may be helpful to 'nest' a person's very specific and personal good life outcomes within nationally recognised outcome frameworks, such as the *Talking Points* framework or *SHANARRI* wellbeing indicators.[10, 11]

Working in this way ensures transparency and accountability without restricting the flexibility that is a key component of an ISF. This level of openness and accountability also ensures that people who have been in receipt of support delivered through more

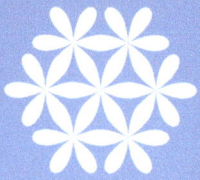

traditional approaches can be assured that their support needs will continue to be met and that they will remain safe and well.

Using an ISF enables more creative solutions. These can often be simple in their application, but life changing in the affect they have on an individual's quality of life.

General Principles:

- An individual budget managed using an ISF should support a good life not just the purchase of a service.
- In a time of reduced funding and increased demand providing the same traditional services with less money is not feasible.
- We need to be prepared to think differently, be creative and consider responses that are not about services.
- Using an ISF, resources can go further by thinking differently. Solutions can be sought that may be simple but make a real difference to people's quality of life.
- The use of money from the budget must be clearly related to the outcomes specific to the person and their plan. It is helpful, for the purposes of accountability, if these are linked to broader national outcomes frameworks.
- Support planning needs to be clear and transparent, people need to be assured that their support needs will still be met and that they will be safe and well.
- Relatively small creative solutions can have a significant positive impact on a person's quality of life.

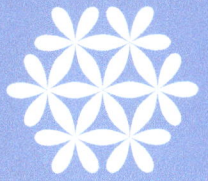

Maria

Maria moved into a congregate living arrangement where she received support during the day and had shared access to a sleepover. She had no idea what her support arrangement cost. Through a process of individualising the service, everyone involved received an individual budget allocation to plan their support. Others in the service decided that they didn't want to contribute towards a sleepover that they didn't need or use. Maria still wanted to access a sleepover.

Using her individual budget allocation, Maria was supported to plan for what she really wanted. When she realised how much of her budget would be required to pay for a sleepover, to be there 'just in case' something happened, she came up with an alternative arrangement that made sense for her. Maria purchased an iPad and negotiated an arrangement with her team that she would Facetime them for half an hour each evening. This proved to be a cost effective creative solution which provided Maria with the reassurance she needed. It also ensured she had money left in her budget to pursue her other goal of setting up a small catering business.

What to expect if you have chosen Option 2 and are using an ISF:

- You are involved in planning and thinking about what a good life means for you.
- You can plan to use your ISF for a wide range of solutions, not just support hours.
- You spend money on things that help you achieve the things in your life you have agreed (outcomes).
- Flexibility ensures that as your life changes, how you use your ISF changes too.
- Your support provider helps you how to work out how to you spend your ISF on other things not just on them.
- You feel listened to and in control.

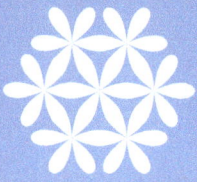

What an organisation must have in place if they are offering ISFs:

- Skill necessary to undertake good creative planning that helps people think about what a good life might look like.
- Necessary time and space to ensure people can consider a wide range of possibilities.
- Flexibility that ensures that a new plan is created as the person's life changes.
- Planning needs to have a direct relationship to the budget
- Capacity to enable the person to use their money for ordinary things and using simple solutions.
- Systems that are transparent and provide regular financial information in a way that is personalised and makes sense to the person.

What commissioners must have in place if they are funding an ISF:

- Clear plans identifying how money will be used to meet the person's agreed outcomes.
- Contracts that enable flexibility so everyday details of individual plans can change in response to life changes, with minimum bureaucracy.
- Ability to support a plan which demonstrates reasonable risk management.
- Transparent personalised accounting system for the ISF relative to the amount of money.

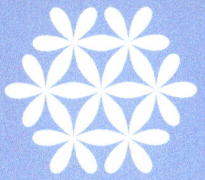

Andrew

Andrew had lengthy experience of institutional support, having entered the care system at the age of eight. He lived in a variety of residential hospitals including the State Hospital Carstairs during which time he acquired a significant reputation for challenging the services that supported him. He eventually moved into a congregate living arrangement (core and cluster) where he shared support with others.

From Andrew's perspective, he experienced greater restrictions and arbitrary rules in the community placement than in hospital. The service was block funded. A new provider took over the service following a tender process and individualised the funding and introduced ISFs.

Andrew took greater control over his life and the decisions he was making. He organised his support in a way that made sense for him. As a consequence, Andrew no longer needs to 'challenge' anyone to have his voice heard. Within 3 years he successfully applied to be removed from all compulsory measures (Guardianship and Compulsory Treatment Order).

Andrew is newly married and is living his 'good life' with his wife Theresa. He uses his ISF to get support around the things that he still finds a little tricky, mostly managing his money and household budgets.

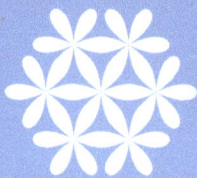

4. Maximum control

Having an individual budget gives a person the opportunity to have a greater say over the support they receive. Having a Direct Payment ensures that they have control over how their individual budget is used. ISFs offer the opportunity to broaden the scope of who can enjoy this level of choice, control and self-direction, beyond those who want to take on the full responsibility for managing a Direct Payment. Not everyone wants to, or can, oversee all aspects of managing an individual budget and support. ISFs enable people to choose the level of involvement they want to have, including how much or how little they want to be involved in managing their budget and support arrangement.

Whatever level of involvement a person agrees, this should not be fixed, it should be routinely reviewed and may change over time. For example, some individuals have opted to manage their money using an ISF and then move on to taking a Direct Payment when circumstances were more stable and they felt more confident. Alternatively, individuals have taken a Direct Payment and then, when circumstances changed, asked for it to be managed through an ISF. Figure 3 illustrates the flow of accountability associated with a Direct Payment and an ISF.

The inbuilt flexibility of an ISF means that, should unforeseen events occur and the level of support required to manage the budget and support increases, the ISF should flex to accommodate the changes required. Ideally an ISF offers all the choice and control of a Direct Payment without the need to take on the full responsibility for managing a budget or becoming an employer. In this respect, the flexibility of an ISF is the key to opening the opportunity for more people to direct their support using Option 2.

There is a significant level of accountability built into the functioning of an ISF. If a person is unable to make decisions about how their budget is spent, they can still have an ISF managed for them but it must be clear who is making decisions on their behalf. Support organisations are often placed in the role of being the decision-maker for people who may lack capacity and have no family or friends, this is not a new

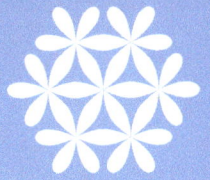

situation and providers can and do act with integrity. However, it must be recognised that if someone has no one in their life to help them plan or make decisions, other than paid support, the priority in their support plan must be to address this issue through cultivating friendships, developing a circle of support or accessing independent advocacy. Statutory services have a clear role in ensuring that there are no concerns over damaging or unhelpful conflicts of interest and third party supports should be accessed if any concerns arise.

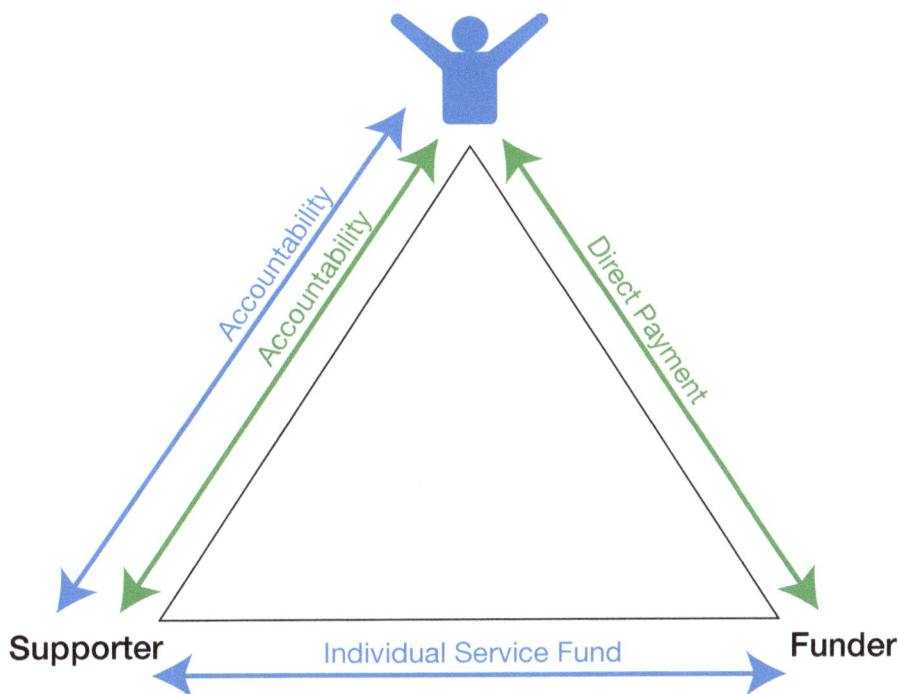

FIGURE 3. ACCOUNTABILITY

ISFs ensure that individuals, or those closest to them, know and understand the implications of the decisions they are making around the use of their individual budget. It enables thinking and planning around the rhythms and patterns of everyday life rather than the fixed patterns and structures of 'serviceland'. The focus on decision making sitting with, or as close to the person as possible, ensures that plans and actions are real, relevant and effective, drawing on the dreams

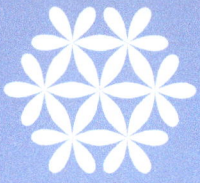

and aspirations of the person at the centre of the plan. This approach draws on the individual agency of the person and those who know them best. It enables incremental developments which can realise transformational change.

General Principles:

- Individual Service Funds are the key to ensuring Self-Directed Support is available to as many people as possible regardless of how involved they can be or want to be in the decision-making process.

- People can choose what parts of their service design, support and budget they want to be in control of or manage and this can be negotiated and change over time.

- People can have all the benefits of Self-Directed Support using an ISF without taking the responsibility for managing the budget or being an employer.

- If the person is not able to make decisions, they can still have an ISF managed for them but it must be clear who is making decisions on their behalf.

- Support organisations are often in the role of being the decision-maker for people who lack capacity and have no family or friends. This is not a new situation and providers can and do act with integrity.

- The ISF planning process offers greater transparency and clarity about who is making decisions on the persons' behalf if needed.

- If a person has no one in their life to help them or make decisions, the priority in their support plan must be to achieve this by for example, consciously creating opportunities for friendships to flourish, actively developing a circle of support.

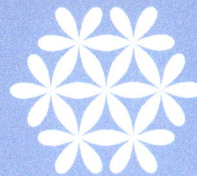

Harriet

Harriet was receiving support from a support organisation, Provider A, but was not happy. She asked to be considered for a Direct Payment but the funder refused. She was advised if she did not like her current provider she should find another one that would directly contract with the local authority. Harriet and her family found Provider B who set up her budget using an ISF. Harriet had as much control as she wanted over her budget and support arrangement.

Several years later Provider B was no longer on the local authority framework. Harriet was advised that she would have to change support provider. Instead Harriet applied for a Direct Payment and this time was successful. Harriet still manages her Direct Payment using her ISF, still supported by Provider B.

The care manager has a role in ensuring there is no concern over unhelpful or damaging conflict of interest and a third party can be used if needed i.e. a broker, a trust, advocacy agency.

What to expect if you have chosen Option 2 and are using an ISF:

- Your planning process includes discussions about how you make decisions in relation to your service and your budget.
- You are clearly able to influence how the plan develops right from the start and can be involved in all the things you want to be i.e. recruiting your own staff.
- Your plan states how you make decisions or who will help you do this.
- A Guardianship order can be applied for if decisions are being made about your welfare on your behalf, but this is not necessary for an ISF to operate.
- You are being offered help, support or information to help you take control and make more decisions.

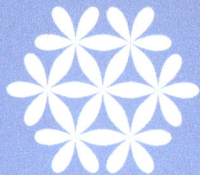

What an organisation must have in place if they are offering ISFs:

- Good planning processes which explicitly detail how the person is involved in decision-making.

- Clear ways the person can be in control and make decisions about their ISF and how it is used for them.

- Flexible processes which enable people to be involved as much as they want to be, e.g. people have a personalised advert and recruitment process.

- The person has a voice and can influence decisions about who works with them, how and when e.g. using a third-party agreement in employment contracts, or how money is spent from their budget.

- Focus on encouraging a wide network of unpaid and paid people to be involved in the person's life.

- Support to involve of independent advocates if the person wants or need them to advocate on their behalf.

- Flexibility, so power and control can move towards the person as they are able and want to take more.

- Simple and easily understood policy and guidance about how to deal with unhelpful or damaging conflicts of interest.

What commissioners must have in place if they are funding an ISF:

- Clarity about how decisions are made and by whom.

- Sensible systems to help explore conflicts of interest without undue bureacracy.

- Care managers or other professionals have a role in ensuring that decisions are made based upon the persons will and preferences.

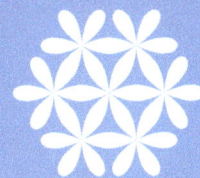

William

William is autistic and had lived in a residential school for most of his teenage years, returning to his family home for holidays and at the weekends. Following school, his family who are also his legal guardians, wanted him to return to their local community where he was well known and connected. William initially wanted to return to the family home full time. With social work support, William's family chose a support provider to work with the whole family to plan his move to the first home of his own.

An individual budget was identified and planning was done. A service design was drawn up by the family and the provider and ISF was established to manage William's individual budget. With support from the provider the family recruited William's team. William's support revolves around his family and other life commitments and changes on a day to day week to week basis. The provider reports to the family about the spend on his budget and they work together to ensure that decisions reflect William's will and preferences.

William has settled in to his home and can now tell people, including his family, when he would like some private time and that he would like them to go. He is able to express choice and control over how he lives his life and his support arrangement will change with him as he flourishes.

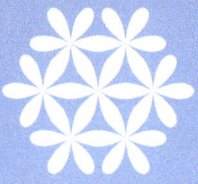

Conclusion

The full impact of the Social Care (Self-Directed Support) (Scotland) Act 2013 has yet to be realised. ISFs offer the opportunity for this groundbreaking legislation to have a positive impact on the lives of far more citizens of Scotland. ISFs are the key to unlocking the potential for a greater number of people to experience choice and control over the support they require to lead a good and meaningful life.

Independent living is the 'North Star' to which Self-Directed Support orients. Direct Payments, hard fought for by disabled people, offer the opportunity to take an individual budget and employ Personal Assistants; an arrangement that provides the greatest level of choice and control over how support is arranged and managed.

With this option however, comes the responsibility for directly employing PAs, and whilst there is good support available to assist with this, not everyone is willing or able to take on this level of responsibility.[12]

By selecting Option 2 of the Act and opting for an ISF, individuals can negotiate the level of involvement they want to have in the management of their budget and support arrangement. Importantly this can and should change over time as life circumstances change.

This paper outlines the core components of an ISF and provides some simple questions that may help individuals, families providers and funders navigate the often bewildering world of social care. The lived examples reveal how simple solutions often bring about transformational change. At their best, ISFs offer the opportunity for decision making to remain by or as close to the person as possible, ensuring that choice and control over the support a person receives is available to the many, not just the few.

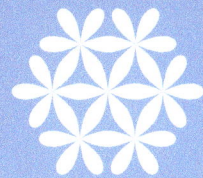

Endnotes

1. United Nations (2006) *Convention on the Rights of Persons with Disabilities.* Treaty Series Vol 2515 P 3

2. *Council of Europe, European Convention for the Protection of Human Rights and Fundamental Freedoms, as amended by Protocols Nos. 11 and 14, 4 November 1950*

3. www.gov.scot/Publications/2015/02/9966/9

4. Fair Work Convention (2016) *Fair Work Framework.* Glasgow: Fair Work Directorate.

5. The Scottish Government (2104) *Statutory guidance to accompany the Social care (Self-Directed Support) (Scotland) Act 2013.* Edinburgh, The Scottish Government.

6. Scottish Executive (2003) *A Guide to receiving Direct Payments in Scotland.* Edinburgh: Scottish Executive.

7. Animate (2014) Individual Service Funds - Learning from Inclusion's 18 years of practice. Sheffield: Centre for Welfare Reform.

8. Partners for Inclusion and C-Change Scotland (formerly C-Change for Inclusion) have operated ISFs since their inception in 2001.

9. see note 5.

10. www.gov.scot/Topics/Health/Quality-Improvement-Performance/Joint-Improvement-Team

11. www.gov.scot/Topics/People/Young-People/gettingitright/wellbeing

12. see *Glasgow Centre for Inclusive Living* www.gcil.org.uk and *Scottish Personal Assistant Employers Network* www.spaen.co.uk

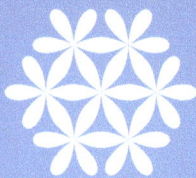

Further reading

Animate (2014) *Individual Service Funds – Learning from Inclusion's 18 years of practice.* Sheffield: Centre for Welfare Reform.

Audit Scotland (2017) *Self-Directed Support 2017 Progress Report.* Edinburgh: Audit Scotland.

Duffy S (2013) Travelling Hopefully - best practice in self-directed support. Sheffield: Centre for Welfare Reform.

Duffy S (2006) Keys to Citizenship: A guide to getting good support for people with learning disabilities, second revised edition. Sheffield: Centre for Welfare Reform.

Duffy S & Sly S (2017) Progress on Personalised Support - results of an international survey by Citizen Network. Sheffield: Centre for Welfare Reform.

Ellis R, Sines D & Hogard E (2014) Better Lives. Sheffield: Centre for Welfare Reform.

Fitzpatrick J (2010) Personalised Support: How to provide high quality support to people with complex and challenging needs - learning form Partners for Inclusion. Sheffield: Centre for Welfare Reform.

Hyde C (2012) Freedom Fighters. Kilmarnock: Partners for Inclusion.

In Control Scotland (2014) *Testing out Individual Service Funds and spending a budget flexibly - An independent evaluation of the NHS Highland Individual Service Fund trial November 2013- April 2014* Glasgow: In Control Scotland.

Iriss Pilotlight *Accessible Information Guide to Individual Service Funds (two-way contract)*: http://pilotlight.iriss.org.uk/resources/accessible-information-guide-individual-service-fund-two-way-contract

Kettle M (2015) *Self-Directed Support - an exploration of Option 2 in practice* Glasgow: Glasgow Caledonian University/P&P.

Sly S & Tindall B (2016) Citizenship: a guide for providers of support. Sheffield: Centre for Welfare Reform.

Social Services Knowledge Scotland http://www.ssks.org.uk/topics/self-directed-support.aspx

Thistle Foundation (2015) *I would never have believed... Learning from the Individual service Fund pilot 2014* Edinburgh: Thistle Foundation.

TLAP (2015) Individual Service Funds (ISFs) and Contracting for Flexible Support. London: TLAP.

WAIS (2012) Shared Management. Perth: WAIS.

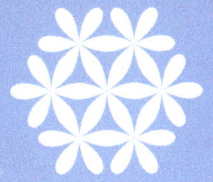

About the authors

Sam Smith

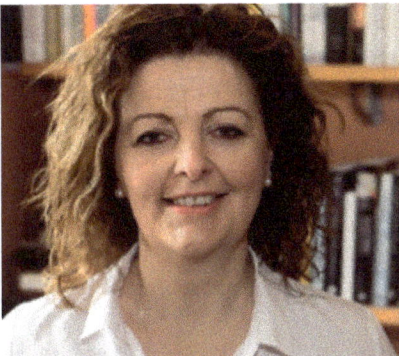

Dr Sam Smith is the founder and CEO of C-Change Scotland, a not for profit organisation supporting disabled people to live the lives they choose. Sam also writes and campaigns on issues of human rights, equality and social justice. Sam's book *Human Rights and Social Care: Putting rights into practice* will be published in May 2018.

Sam offers consultancy in organisational development, creative service design, inclusive practice, individual budgets and human rights. Drawing on academic theory and extensive practical experience Sam is both an informative and charismatic public speaker.

Email: sam.smith@c-change.org.uk

Website: www.c-change.org.uk

Frances Brown

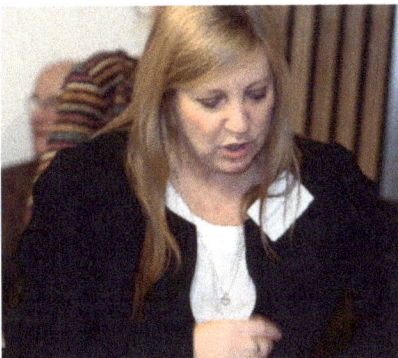

Frances's background is in mental health and learning disability nursing. She has worked for the NHS and a range of third sector organisations in Scotland and was previously the Director of Inclusion Glasgow. Frances was one of the joint development officers of In Control Scotland.

Frances now works as an independent consultant specialising in self-directed support and service design and is joint founder of the consultancy Radical Visions.

Email: francesbrown1960@gmail.com

Website: www.radicalvisions.wpengine.com

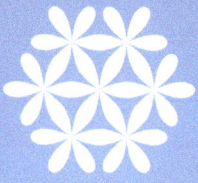

In Control Scotland

In Control Scotland supports the successful implementation of self-directed support in Scotland by working with and alongside people and organisations. We are involved in providing a range of events, activities, information and opportunities to share practice and experiences so that people can take control, make choices and live the life they want.

To find out more go to www.in-controlscotland.org

To join our mailing list for news and events email: info@in-controlscotland.org.uk

Centre for Welfare Reform

The Centre for Welfare Reform is an independent think tank. Its aim is to transform the current welfare state so that it supports citizenship, family and community. It works by developing and sharing social innovations and influencing government and society to achieve necessary reforms.

To find out more go to www.centreforwelfarereform.org

We produce a monthly email newsletter, if you would like to subscribe to the list please visit: bit.ly/CfWR-subscribe

Follow us on twitter: @CforWR

Find us on Facebook: fb.me/centreforwelfarereform

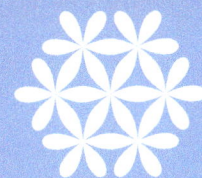

Citizen Network

This guide has been published in association with Citizen Network, an international movement to achieve citizenship for all. Citizen Network brings together all those around the world who want to overcome prejudice, poverty and powerlessness.

We believe in diversity and equality: every single individual is equal and our differences are something to be acknowledged, nurtured and celebrated.

Anyone or any group who believes in these values can join Citizen Network.

People with disabilities, particularly people with more complex needs or people with mental health problems, too often find themselves stripped of their status as citizens. They are excluded, placed in institutional hospitals, care homes or special unit, cut off from their family, friends and community. This is not just an abuse of human rights, it is a serious loss to all of us. We all belong and we must work together to ensure that everyone gets the chance to have a life of meaning, freedom and contribution.

Find out more about Citizen Network, and please join us:

Visit: www.citizen-network.org

Follow us on twitter: @citizen_network

Find us on facebook: fb.me/citizennetwork

www.ingramcontent.com/pod-product-compliance
Lightning Source LLC
Chambersburg PA
CBHW061012030426
42336CB00028B/3454